GW00480500

Royalties from this book will be donated entirely to
Animal Free Research UK
animalfreeresearchuk.org
Animal Free Research UK is a registered charity in England and
Wales (No. 1146896) and Scotland (No. SC045327) and a company
limited by guarantee in England and Wales (No. 08015625).
Registered Office: 27 Old Gloucester Street, London, WC1N 3AX

Steven Liska

How Life Can Change

At A Stroke

or

"A Life Turned Upside Down"

Linda was a normal, healthy,
hard-working mother of two
when at the age of 56
she was seriously disabled in an instant
by a massive stroke.

This is her story
with locations as diverse as Hertfordshire,
Bohemia, the Isle of Man and Wales
…and quite a few lovely dogs.

TABLE OF CONTENTS

Chapter 1 - Bohemian Like You *7*

Chapter 2 - Let's Get Together *15*

Chapter 3 - What's Going On? *23*

Chapter 4 - The Shape I'm In *29*

Chapter 5 - Starting Over *39*

Chapter 6 - Help! *51*

Chapter 7 - Learning to Fly *61*

Chapter 8 - Get 'em Out By Friday *73*

Chapter 9 - You Made Me A Nervous Wreck *78*

Chapter 10 - Ain't No Sunshine *85*

Chapter 11 - Let's Get Married *91*

Chapter 12 - A Design For Life *99*

Chapter 13 - Deeply Dippy *121*

Chapter 14 - I Don't Wanna Talk About It *127*

Chapter 15 - Synchronicity *139*

Chapter 16 - Drive *157*

Chapter 17 - Carry On *165*

Acknowledgements *175*

CHAPTER 1

BOHEMIAN LIKE YOU

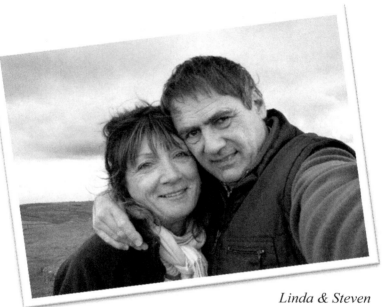

*Linda & Steven
at Bungalow,
Isle of Man TT course, 2007*

This is the story of a medical stroke, and of its many consequences. It's not really written as an entertainment but hopefully it'll be informing and enlightening (and that you'll like the pictures). It's about an incident that took place at the end of 2011, the repercussions of which are still ongoing. I guess I should tell you the cast of characters first.

I'm Steven, and I lived in the Hertfordshire village of Chipperfield when, in 2007, I 'virtually' met Linda, who lived a few miles away in Welwyn Garden City. We wrote to each other for some time and so got to know each other pretty well before finally getting together one evening at Verulam Park in St. Albans. Linda's marriage had failed and none of my previous relationships had reached extra time either. Music was an early bond, and we were soon bringing songs to the relationship, mine was 'Bohemian like you' by the Dandy Warhols, and Linda's was 'Nice weather for ducks' by Lemon jelly.

My mother had died in 2005 and almost immediately my dad, who I was increasingly caring for, was diagnosed with prostate cancer. Happily though, he was still in fine form in 2007 and along with my little rescue dog Lucy, we all went off to the Norfolk coast on holiday for a few days so Linda got to know Dad pretty well. He was already 90 years old but the illness didn't start to bite until the spring/summer of 2008.

Whilst in Great Yarmouth I scattered my Mum's ashes at the Parish Church opposite the White Horse Inn, which her Mum used to run in the fifties and sixties, and off the harbour's mouth where they both loved to watch the ships come and go in times gone by.

Later on, I took Linda and Lucy on the Manx ferry for a week to the Isle of Man. A bit late in the year, so no racing or rallying to enjoy, but plenty of sightseeing and visiting of old friends to pass the time.

I got to know Linda's two boys, Alex and Dan, and we got to know each other more. Early on she realised 'there will always be a dog', and whilst not being used to their company, she soon came to love and appreciate Lucy, who came almost everywhere on holidays with us, most of them being to Wales or the Isle of Man. Linda would spend weekends with me and I'd visit her home in Welwyn Garden City during the week.

Sometimes we'd meet up for gigs at the University of Hertfordshire in Hatfield, where she worked, on one occasion emailing me asking "Have you ever heard of this chap?". He turned out to be James Litherland, one time guitarist with supergroup Colosseum, one of my favourite bands, and he signed one of my albums that night.

Gradually Dad's condition deteriorated as the cancer metastasised and spread to his spine, and I did all I could to make him comfortable at home but one Saturday night in September he was so bad I couldn't lift him and had to ask for the ambulance to attend. The crew, perhaps not surprisingly, didn't think that taking him to A&E in Watford on a Saturday night was a very good idea so they helped me to get him settled.

The next morning however I found him collapsed across the bed and it became obvious that he needed full time professional care and I managed to get him into the hospice in Berkhamsted, where he passed on only ten days later.

Linda came all the way over from Welwyn to be with me and Lucy that full moon Monday night, and was a great support for me.

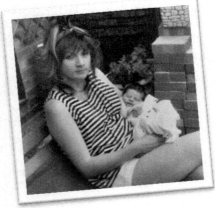

*Linda
with baby Alex*

*Linda with her sons
Danny & Alex*

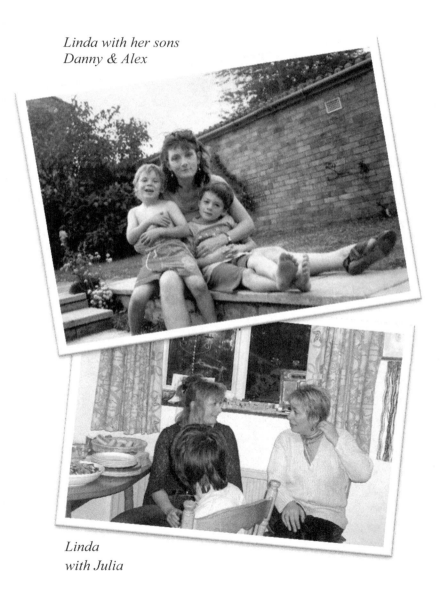

*Linda
with Julia*

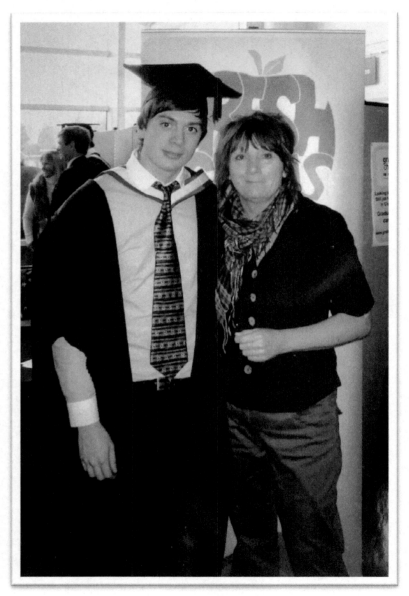

Linda at Alex's graduation

CHAPTER 2

LET'S GET TOGETHER

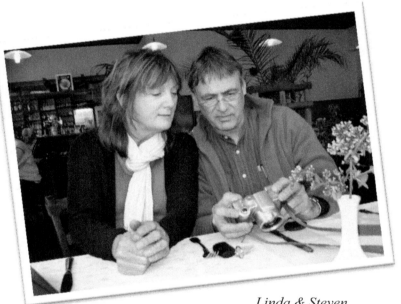

Linda & Steven,
viewing photos from
Dad's Memorial Service,
Czech Republic 2010

Gradually life settled down into a new pattern, with me continuing to work on cars at home and us spending even more time with each other. Linda's mum Olive was also becoming progressively more ill, and Linda was spread very thin with her commitments so we tried to help each other as much as we could.

We also found time to get away as much as possible though, after Dad passed in September 2008, we spent a week on the west coast of the Isle of Man. The next year we flew to Portugal for a week and managed to see some of the World Championship Rally of Portugal. At other times we visited just about every part of Wales, staying variously at Tenby, Broadhaven, Cardigan, Llandudno and the Llyn peninsula, during which trip we went to Llanberis. Linda climbed Snowdon on a pretty hot day and reported that coming down was worse than going up.

We also drove all the way to the Czech Republic in 2010 to take Dad's ashes back to the family grave in Bohemia, though Lucy stayed in Chipperfield this time with my friend Margy Bruin.

Winter 2011 was setting in and whilst I'd become a registered pet sitter and had been looking after dogs at home as well as fixing cars, I had no dog boarders on Sunday the 11th December, just a Volvo that I'd been working on in the garage. Linda meanwhile was doing some 'homework', (for her job as an admin at Hertfordshire University) on the laptop that evening. It was all to no avail however, the work she did that evening never made it back to her office.

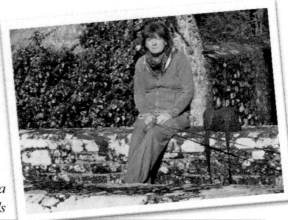

Linda at St. Davids

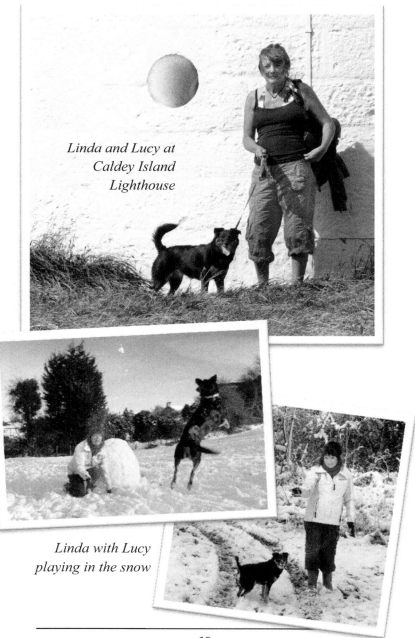

Linda and Lucy at Caldey Island Lighthouse

Linda with Lucy playing in the snow

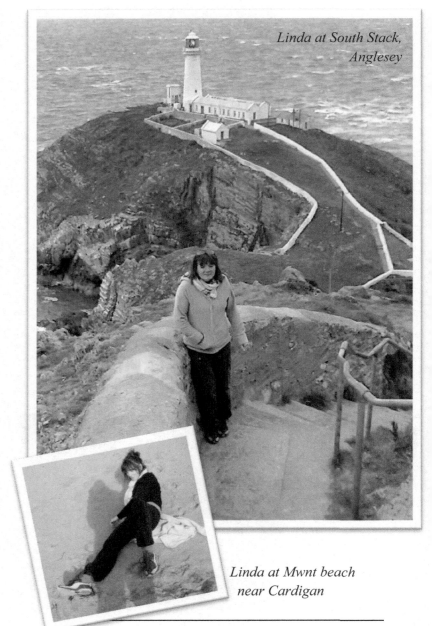

Linda at South Stack, Anglesey

Linda at Mwnt beach near Cardigan

*Linda, Lucy and a well-preserved Suzuki 250,
Manx Grand Prix*

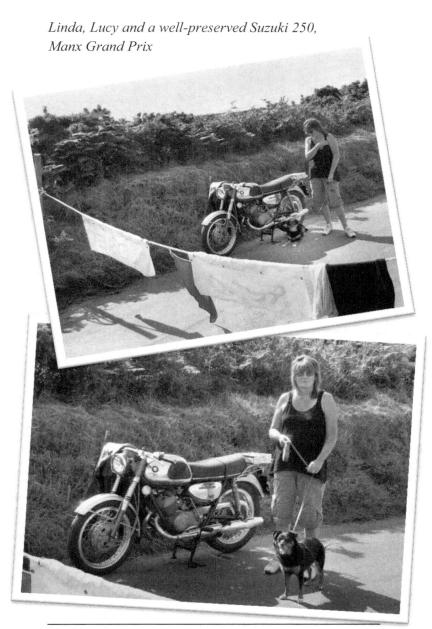

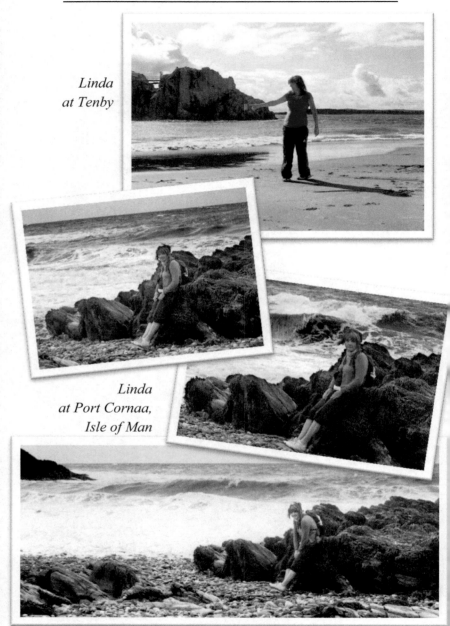

*Linda
at Tenby*

*Linda
at Port Cornaa,
Isle of Man*

CHAPTER 3

WHAT'S GOING ON?

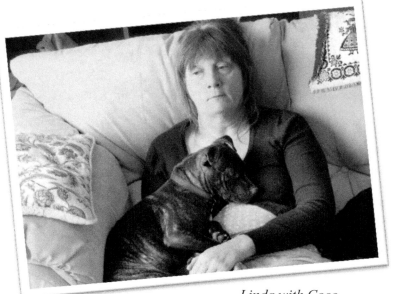

Linda with Coco
(1st image after her stroke)

On the morning of December 12th, Linda was due to return early from Chipperfield to her home in Welwyn Garden City to meet a workman who had a job to do in the house. At 7.45 she did indeed wake up, and woke me with her, by making strange and worrying noises that made no sense in the grey light of dawn. I apologised as I turned on the bedroom light to try and make more sense of what I was hearing, and soon realised that she was ill, very ill.

This seemed completely illogical at the time, she was fit, strong, swam and walked regularly, and worked more than full time to keep everything together with job, family and relationships, but as I asked her more questions which went unanswered, I finally said "If you don't answer the next question, I'm calling the ambulance". Well, she didn't, and I did, and despite living in a rural location I must say that help turned up remarkably quickly and the 999 operator stayed on the line to help me while we were waiting.

Inevitably I was asked about animals in the house and had to shut Lucy in the living room lest the ambulance crew tripped over her, aside from that she would merely have licked them all over. I discussed with the operator what might be going on, I think I already had a hunch that it was a stroke but even the paramedics seemed to be unsure, they actually called Linda 'an enigma'.

They took Linda away to Watford general, about twenty to thirty minutes away and I tried to come up with a suitable plan of action. First, I had to find someone to take care of Lucy, and Margy Bruin was the natural choice. She lived nearby on the edge of the woods on Chipperfield Common and I trusted her completely. Luckily, she answered my call and was ready when I took Lucy to her house.

Then I had to call the boys, and let them know what had happened, and also the owner of the Volvo I'd been working on, who thankfully wasn't in too great a hurry for its return.

The boys admitted that if their Mum had the stroke at home, they probably wouldn't have known at the time. They'd have most likely left for work without checking on her knowing that she was waiting in for the visitor.

Then I set off for Vicarage Road, Watford, not on this occasion to watch my favourite team, but to find out more about Linda's condition. As I remember, there was a ward behind A&E with subdued lighting, and Linda lying in bed before being transferred to the stroke ward upstairs. It seems that she had already been scanned and thrombo-lysed as it was apparent that the stroke was not a bleed but a blood clot, and the drugs she'd been given were an attempt to dissolve the clot and mitigate the damage.

She was not very responsive and I had to wait until she'd been settled in the stroke ward and arrange for the boys to visit. The first ward she was in yet again had a somewhat subdued atmosphere, but within a week or so she'd been transferred to a much brighter environment and had a bed by the window, overlooking an area called The Rookery, well known to fans of Watford FC.

The football club is right next door to the hospital and when she was well enough, I'd take her in a wheelchair for night-time magical mystery tours and end up looking out over the stadium and the bright lights of Watford. Not the most thrilling view in the world but at least she was up and about and starting to connect with the outside world again.

Linda with Freddie, Jack and Lucy

CHAPTER 4

THE SHAPE I'M IN

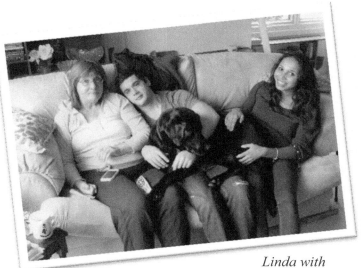

*Linda with
Danny, Lois & Theo*

The diagnosis had been made, she'd experienced Atrial Fibrillation, a condition she was unaware of, despite being on medication for high blood pressure. I do wonder why she hadn't been more thoroughly checked for such a condition, knowing there was an issue with blood pressure, though I believe it's not always possible to predict. The AF had temporarily stopped her heart, allowing the blood to start to coagulate and form a clot, which upon the heart restarting had been propelled into the left side of the brain. The result was paralysis of her dominant right side, particularly her hand and arm, partial paralysis of the right leg, and worst of all, loss of most of her speech and ability to read and write. In technical terms she'd suffered a 'left total anterior circulation infarct', apparently infarction is the process that causes the damage, in this case ischemic necrosis, and infarct is the damage thus caused.

Both of Linda's brothers are left-handed, and now she is as well. She has learnt over the years to write simple words and phrases with her left hand and can understand some familiar words as well, but she has completely lost the ability to read a book, or even a line of subtitles on the TV. She's never really taken to audio books either and while I try to read to her at times, it doesn't seem to work very well or be a satisfactory alternative to her own ability to read.

Six weeks passed in the stroke ward, with gradual rehabilitation efforts being started. The physio room was right next door and I happened to be there one day when she was being encouraged to walk again and one of the physios was unduly impatient with her. I was upset enough to complain about it, knowing full well that she was making every effort to improve her condition, and what she'd been through already. Just for the record she underwent another ECG on the 27th of February and wore a heart monitor for a while as well.

I took a book along to show to Linda, 'My Championship Year', the story of Jenson Button's Formula One World Championship in 2009. I love Motorsport and as well as the few stages of the Rally of Portugal we'd seen in 2009 we had also seen a couple of Manx Grand Prix together on the Isle of Man but had not got into the habit of watching F1 on a regular basis.

I thought the wonderful colour photos in the book would help to brighten her up and distract her from the pretty awful situation she found herself in. She was now unable to read, something she loved, and virtually unable to speak so was locked in to a great extent and anything I could do to cheer her up was worth trying. We now watch all the Grand Prix races we can and not surprisingly Hertfordshire born Lewis Hamilton is our favourite, along with Mexican driver Sergio Perez. One evening I brought a little treat into the ward for her and the lady in the bed opposite - a small gin and tonic each. One nurse told us off by stating that it was alcohol that had caused the stroke, which was completely untrue. I thought this a very unkind and unnecessary intrusion.

The two young lady doctors that attended to Linda were very pleasant however and her sons and brother Gary, as well as her ex-husband John also visited. John's sister Julia is married to a now retired GP, Charles, and they also visited from their home in Willesden, Charles providing more insight into Linda's medical condition. He told us that when he was training at St. Thomas' hospital in the seventies, stroke patients were stuck at the end of the ward and received very little help with rehabilitation and recovery. He was pleasantly surprised that Watford had a dedicated stroke ward, I won't tell you what he said about the car parking though, this is a family story.

The week after Linda's stroke, one of my neighbours in Chipperfield, the farmer John Saunders also had a stroke and ended up in an adjoining ward - something in the water, or the air? Luckily his stroke was nowhere near as severe and his speech was unaffected and, as far as I know, the only lingering disability was to one of his arms.

Christmas was approaching, as well as my sixtieth birthday on the 27th, and my friend Tine, who lives near the hospital, put me up one evening after visiting time. Then I travelled up to Willesden to stay with Charles and Julia, visiting Linda as well of course. I think it was the morning of my birthday, whilst in the kitchen, that I heard a commotion upstairs and went up to see Lucy, and Charles and Julia's dog Billie, pinned in a corner of the landing by an angry looking cat that belonged to Sophie, the youngest daughter of the household who was visiting from Brighton.

When I told my sister she asked "What was the cat's name, Wellard?" Lucy was no shrinking violet herself, but luckily the three must have come to some sort of agreement about territorial rights...

So, another month passed while treatment continued and after six weeks, on January 25th, Linda was transferred to a rehabilitation unit at Old Welwyn, only a couple of miles from her home. There she spent two months, undergoing more therapy and eventually moving from a single room with bathroom to more of a self-contained flat where she could practice some simple domestic tasks as well.

One advantage of the rehab unit was that I could take Lucy in to see Linda. One evening we walked in and I was challenged by a nurse who very forcefully told me that dogs weren't allowed. "Yes they are" I told her, "I checked with the manager" and kept on going.

I would take Lucy around the grounds and into the common rooms as well where she was warmly welcomed by the patients.

I was concerned that Linda wasn't receiving much in the way of speech therapy, and one day I copied the list of treatment sessions, here it is…

	MON	TUE	WED	THU	FRI
09:00		Occu-pational	Occu-pational	Occu-pational	Occu-pational
09:30		Therapy	Therapy	Therapy	Therapy
10:00		Upper Limb	Physio		Baking Group
10:30	Upper Limb				
11:00		Physio			
11:30					Core Group
12:00			Lunch Break		
13:00					
13:30				Physio	
14:00		Speech			
14:30				Upper Limb	
15:00	Physio				
15:30		OT	Upper Limb		
16:00	Speech				
16:30					
17:00					

The schedule always seemed light on speech therapy to me. I know that stroke victims need a lot of rest, but only two sessions a week didn't appear to do much to address the worst aspect of the stroke (as far as we were concerned) - the lack of speech.

The 'flat' was also, strangely, rather dark and gloomy and I was glad when she was allowed to leave. Of course, she couldn't go back to her house and her old life, so I asked her to come and live with me in Chipperfield so I could look after her and so from the spring of 2012 to the summer of 2014 life's pattern changed completely.

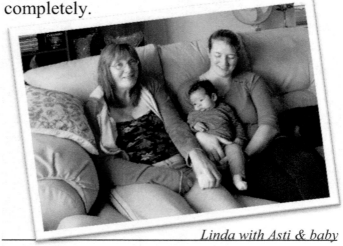

Linda with Asti & baby

CHAPTER 5

STARTING OVER

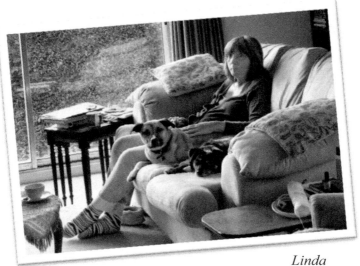

Linda
with Rio & Lucy

I was still able to work on some cars but with Linda now at home full time I was better able to do as a job what in hindsight I should have done all my life, look after dogs and other animals. I'm convinced that the company of so many lovely dogs was very comforting for Linda as well.

Someone once asked me where the kennels were. "They sleep on the bed if they want to"' I told them, "or anywhere else they like". Kennels indeed! It was their home as long as they were with us and Lucy welcomed them all as well. We only had two or three boarders at most at any one time and somehow, we got by financially even though two of my neighbours were causing a great many problems. At least one neighbour, a lovely Welshman, was very supportive and kind and helped us a great deal but eventually we decided to sell the house and move away completely.

My first choice was the Isle of Man, but Linda thought this was too far away for the boys to be able to visit so the second choice was probably more sensible in terms of facilities that would be available to help her recovery.

In the summer of 2013, we stayed at a lovely house in Dwygyfylchi, (pronunciation lessons available on request) near to Conwy and Llandudno.

Exactly 100 years before in 1913, Sir Edward Elgar had stayed at this house, 'Tan yr Allt', or Under the Hill, for several months and had finished writing his Falstaff suite there. Elgar being one of the very few classical composers that I like, this was added inducement and to see what he had seen 100 years ago, (minus the A55 dual carriageway), was particularly evocative. Beautiful views across the sea to Anglesey, Puffin Island, and, to the North, the Great Orme at Llandudno.

So it was that on the 21st March 2012, a lovely sunny day, Linda came home to my bungalow 'Rosemary' and it was all change again, we didn't really need modifications to the house but we did get a bath board for Linda to sit on while I showered her, as I remember that was all that we needed at first. However, she had always used contact lenses but could no longer fit them herself so I took her down to the opticians in Chesham for an eye test and glasses, thankfully her eyesight wasn't affected, even though that can be a consequence of stroke.

This brings to mind one of the practical problems that arose, in that previously Linda had used Boots Opticians for her contact lenses, but I didn't know this. To their great credit they sent a lovely hand-written letter offering to help her with the backlog of orders and the direct debits and expressing hope for her recovery. I still don't know how they knew that she'd been ill, and now that she couldn't speak, I was not even aware that she used Boots in Hatfield, but I was very pleased and im-pressed that their staff were so thoughtful.

There were even bigger problems to come regarding her bank account with the Co-op and her mobile phone account with Virgin, as she hadn't written down any passwords or any other details.

Managers from the University of Hertfordshire, where Linda worked, became involved as it was obvious now that she would not be able to return to work anytime soon, if at all. We were visited by them at home and we also went to the University for a medical assessment in May.

As well as getting used to the treatment rota we also took on a new drug regime, here's another list for you…

Medication	Dosage per day
Simvastatin 40mg	1x
Citalopram 10mg	1x
Lansoprazole 15mg	1x
Fludrocortisone 100µg	1x
Amitriptyline 20mg	1x
Codeine 30 mg x up to 4	1x
Paracetamol 1g	up to 4x

Oh, I nearly forgot! Warfarin!
Dose dependent on the International
Normalized Ratio (INR) - a measure of
how long it takes for blood to clot in a
sample. This, for several years, meant
regular visits to the GP for testing and
dosing, but since we moved to Wales,
we've obtained our own machine to test the
INR and we let the surgery know the
reading and they then call back with the
appropriate dose.

The Amitriptyline was prescribed for
thalamic pain/central post-stroke pain
which can occur after stroke involving
damage to the thalamus. Luckily this
specific type of pain doesn't seem to have
occurred, although reading the list of
symptoms that can result from damage to
the thalamus is pretty frightening, and not
surprisingly include impaired motor
function, speech and cognition.

On a couple of occasions, we've met
people who have suffered stroke and they

claim to have rid themselves of the worst effects by means of hard work and determination. This seems to be a somewhat arrogant and unkind view that could engender guilt in a survivor who has not experienced such a full recovery. Clearly strokes come in all different shapes and sizes, and implying that a patient has not worked hard enough to overcome the effects is extremely unhelpful.

One of Linda's consultants told us that one in three patients who suffered a stroke of the magnitude of hers would have died, and that the others would have ended up in an institution. It was that bad, and sometime later we attended Bangor University for testing and therapy and a very much more detailed brain scan than the NHS ones she'd had.

We soon obtained a computer software programme called 'StepbyStep' that she could use to try and stimulate her speech and understanding, with help from the

Tavistock Trust for Aphasia. She also started physical and sensory therapy locally at the Herts Neurological service at Abbots Langley, about five miles away. We also had help from an organisation called Speakability, which also supports those with Aphasia/Dysphasia, though why the same condition has two names I never did find out.

Later in the year we had a visit from a co-ordinator at the Stroke association in Watford and as a result Linda started attending the Stroke group in Hemel Hempstead, this took place at the Blind Centre in Boxmoor for two hours every Thursday afternoon.

Now I don't know about you but if I think about those affected by sight loss, I naturally think of Guide dogs so I was amazed to find that dogs were not allowed at these sessions. Luckily the stroke group we eventually attended in Colwyn Bay were happy to accommodate our dogs.

Linda's right hand is virtually paralysed and early on she had a splint specially made to try to alleviate the problem, the hand will grip but not release, and a few different devices were tried over the years to keep it stretched and pliable.

Eventually she started having botox injections in her right arm and right leg to ease the spasticity in the hand and foot muscles and we travel regularly to the hospital at Caernarfon where our lovely Iraqui Doctor Ramadhan and just as lovely Welsh Nurse Caroline administer the very effective treatment which helps to keep things moving. At night in particular, I stretch out and hold Linda's hand to stop it seizing up and also manipulate her right leg and foot with the same aim. The foot is 'dropped' to some extent and twisted to one side so she also uses special shoes with a splint for the right leg.

Back to 2012, Linda had a couple of speech therapy sessions at Hemel Hempstead hospital but yet again they seemed to be too few and too far between and we kept being told that Speech therapy services were being cut back all the time. In April we saw a Specialist Speech and Language Therapist who assessed Linda as "presenting with severe expressive dysphasia with an element of verbal dyspraxia also. She also seems to have a moderate to severe receptive dysphasia characterised by a comprehension level of single written words and one stage spoken commands. I have arranged to see Ms. Dowell for 6 weeks of speech and language therapy to specifically target yes/no reliability, encouraging the use of gesture and drilling of functional spoken phrases". These sessions took place at Hemel Hempstead Hospital.

Honey xx

CHAPTER 6

HELP!

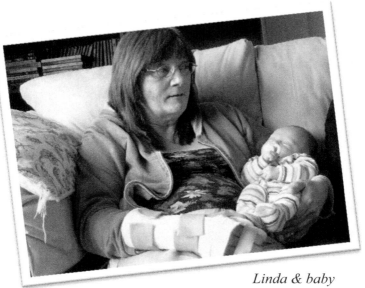

Linda & baby

I was also dealing with the benefits agencies, and one of the most helpful organisations was the Money advice unit at Hertford County Council. I spent two hours talking to them one day while holding the portable phone to my ear with one hand and weeding the garden with the other, they were great.

Contact with the DWP and the Job Centres however was not so easy. This was to make claims for ESA (Employment and Support Allowance) and DLA (Disability Living Allowance). On average, every call to the DWP involves holding on for at least twenty minutes (often more) whilst Vivaldi's four seasons is forced down one ear. I used to quite like the four seasons… Any forms that need filling in involve answering the same questions over and over and over again, most of which they've already been told the answers to.

On one occasion, frustrated by the simplistic and repetitive questions, I decided to go and talk to the Jobcentre in Watford in person. When I got to the address they gave on their forms, in Ascot Road, I found it was a PO Box, and was directed to the Jobcentre in Exchange Road.

When I got there, I found that vehicle access was denied to Joe Public so pleaded my case and was allowed into the car park. How on earth I managed it, I still can't exactly remember but all of a sudden, I was through the hallowed portals and was actually allowed to speak to some of the managers, who to their credit expressed their great sympathy with my plight and all others in the same situation.

It is sadly apparent that none of these agencies will actually tell you what benefits you are entitled to. It's up to you to find out for yourself, whether by luck or persistence, and when you do find out, they will put every obstacle in your way to stop you claiming your legal entitlements.

One of the most irritating questions was along the lines of 'what is your medical condition?' (Possibly the best way to answer it would be a/she's a stroke patient b/she's a stroke survivor c/she's a stroke victim?)

The logical way for me to sum it up is "Well, it's the same as it's been since the massive stroke that the person I'm acting on behalf of experienced it in December 2011. She has not improved since and is almost certainly not going to improve in the future. How do I summarise her medical condition?". "She's in the condition of having suffered a massive stroke, she's half paralysed, to all extents and purposes cannot read or write and will never be able to, she almost certainly won't be able to work again either so please don't expect her to travel to undergo an assessment for work examination".

I must have done something right using this approach because in the final analysis we were not compelled to travel, as so many others had been and probably continue to be, for assessment. If they can't believe expert medical advice they must be clutching at straws. Maybe some people do try it on when claiming benefits, but that's no excuse for tarring everyone with the same brush.

Another trip to Watford was needed to try and sort out Linda's bank account with the Co-op and we didn't get very far without the password as I remember. The manager was very helpful and understanding and probably put a stop on the account but it wasn't until we'd moved to Wales that we finally got the account closed at the branch in Rhyl. Yet again I can't remember how but any such dealings are extremely difficult without all the security details.

The same applied to the mobile phone account with Virgin, who were far less accessible and extremely unhelpful, the less said about them the better. We also applied for a Blue disabled parking badge, more trips to the GP, more forms to fill, more waiting, but eventually it arrived and made trips out a lot easier.

We were happy to see many visitors at 'Rosemary', some of Linda's work colleagues, the boys and their girlfriends, and we had a steady stream of lovely dogs to care for. I have quite a few pictures of Linda cuddling them - Coco the brindle staffie pup, Becky the 20 year-old Yorkie cross, Honey the very old and sweet greyhound who drank tea from our mugs, Rio the staffie cross who climbed trees, Jack the white mongrel and Theo the black lab all from Kings Langley.

We also looked after Billie the Standard Schnauzer for quite a while in the summer, and also loved having Bailey the pointer cross, who was fascinated by shiny little lights and would chase them around the room.

We would take them out for walks on Chipperfield Common or the field by the village hall at Flaunden, or Bovingdon green, and got into a routine quite early whereby I used the walking stick in my left hand and Linda held onto my right arm with her left hand.

All of these fields were quite accessible and all had flat surfaces so were ideal for Linda to practice walking again. As we walked around Flaunden field in particular I would point out the wildflowers in the grass, the buttercups, dandelions, daisies and clover, and ask Linda to repeat the words, she did get better over time but we did get a lot of 'daisycups'. I never knew whether to encourage her to repeat words for practice or not.

I can't help thinking that it must have helped to some extent to keep trying, within reason, to speak again, as long as she didn't get frustrated by the experience.

CHAPTER 7

LEARNING TO FLY

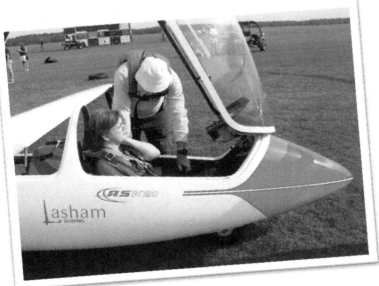

*Linda & Derek
at Lasham*

In September we drove down to Lasham airfield, near Basingstoke in Hampshire and my friend Derek took Linda up for a short flight in a glider. He's a very experienced pilot though sadly the conditions were not good enough that day for a long flight. After getting Linda into the cockpit however (not easy with her disabilities), she thoroughly enjoyed the experience.

I'm always looking for new activities that can help make her life more interesting as losing reading and speech abilities has been pretty devastating for her. On the subject of speech, it may not occur to most people how significant its loss can be. Most people take it for granted that they can communicate without looking at the other party, from a different room, or without looking directly at them, but without speech things change dramatically.

Early on Linda took to calling me by saying 'there', just that, and I knew she was trying to bring my attention to something, the next job was to find out what and that always involves looking directly at each other.

So, if I'm cooking for example and she wants to say something, I have to stop and turn to face her to aid communication and hopefully work out what she wants to tell me. Even then it's not always possible and if she struggles to tell me and I try to guess, it's not long before she gets frustrated and gives up completely.

Sometimes it's a while later that I realise what she was getting at and I can assure you that most communication is NOT non-verbal.

Conveying a simple message like "come here" or "go away" or "I want a drink" might be easy with mime or gesture but try to bring up something abstract like the subject of genealogy or the lyrics of Nick Drake, not so simple.

I asked her if she dreams and what about and she told me that she doesn't dream at all - later amended to dreaming very little, of which she remembers nothing. This seems so sad to me 'cos I dream a lot. I presume this is to do with damage caused by the stroke as well.

Slightly later in the year we went to stay in Llandudno for a few days as we certainly seemed to be focusing our attention on North Wales, having visited pretty well all areas up to that point. We love all of Wales but the North stands out as having the mountains as well as the coast and countryside. It's also closer to Liverpool and therefore to the Manx ferry.

Access is excellent, except to South Wales of course. I guess it's a bit like England in reverse, there you can go up and down with relative ease, sideways is a lot more difficult, whereas in Wales it's not that easy to go anywhere apart from sideways in the North and the South, but it's about four hours to go up or down between the two. The saving grace is of course that it's all incredibly beautiful.

My love affair with Wales started in a small way when a brief detour on the way to Liverpool in 1985 took me through the most beautiful scenery to Lake Vernwy. It carried on in the mid-nineties when a relationship ended and I started travelling to the South. First of all to see where my parents lived in 1942/3, Little Haven in Pembrokeshire, it seemed as good a place to start as anywhere. Dad was an airman with 311 Czech squadron RAF during WW2, first stationed in Norfolk with Bomber command and later on at Talbenny near Haverfordwest on Coastal Command, flying Wellington bombers on anti-submarine sweeps over the Bay of Biscay. He lived nearby at Little Haven with Mum and my sister Anna from late 1942 to mid-1943.

I then learned about the nearby Skokholm and Skomer islands and visited them a few times, actually staying for several nights on Skokholm on two occasions. What a wonderful place to experience close proximity with wild seabirds, Manx shearwaters, Storm Petrels, Puffins etc.

I also got to know Swansea quite well due to my love for the Welsh Prog Rock band 'MAN', who I'd first seen in 1971, supporting 'Argent' at High Wycombe town hall. I fell in love with both bands there and then, but sadly Argent folded a few years later and, though MAN also ceased to be at about the same time, they reformed in the early eighties to carry on delighting ageing hippies everywhere, and hosting their Christmas Parties at the Patti Pavilion in Swansea. These were wonderful events where I also saw the likes of Bonnie Tyler, Trevor Burton (guitarist with The Move), Pete Brown (who wrote many songs for Cream) and the best duo you've never heard of, Gary and Taff, as supporting acts.

In late 2012 and early 2013 life carried on as before with lots of lovely dogs to care for, with Linda carrying on therapy at Jackotsfield rehab centre. There she also took part in a 'Bobarth' course, for the assessment and treatment of adults with neurological conditions. This took a few hours per day for five days in February, but I can't remember any other specific help that we received while we were still in Hertfordshire, other than the regular visits to the stroke group.

So, in June 2013 came our trip to the aforementioned Dwygyfylchi to stay in the Theodosia suite at 'Tan yr Allt'. It's a small self-contained flat that had been built and named for the owner's mother and was now let to visitors. Included in our party were Lucy, of course, and Billie, who was staying with us for a few weeks and naturally came along for the ride.

Whilst there we started looking at properties in the area to get an idea of what we could get and how much we'd need to pay, though one of the attractions of the area was that we would get much more for our money than if we stayed in Hertfordshire. This meant having more income and more spare capacity in case of extra, unforeseen circumstances. However, the main spur was to live near the sea, with the mountains close by, and to have cooler temperatures in the summer and warmer weather in the winter.

I've always struggled in hot weather, by which I mean anything over about 20 centigrade, and although Linda used to enjoy it, she also found the heat too much since the stroke. Locals are surprised when I say that Hertfordshire is hotter in summer and colder in winter but it's true. It's landlocked, and being near the coast in Wales makes all the difference.

We made trips to Anglesey, to see the nesting seabirds at South Stack, into the mountains to Llanberis and Llyn Padarn, around the Great Orme to see the feral Kashmir goats and over the Sychnant pass to see the wild Carneddau mountain ponies.

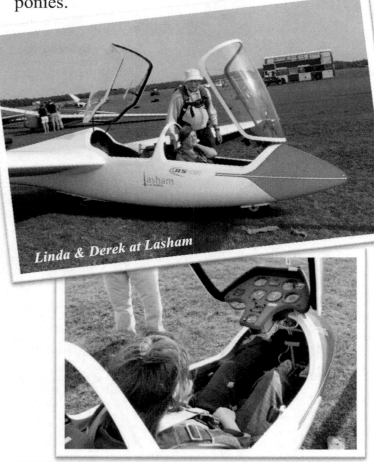

Linda & Derek at Lasham

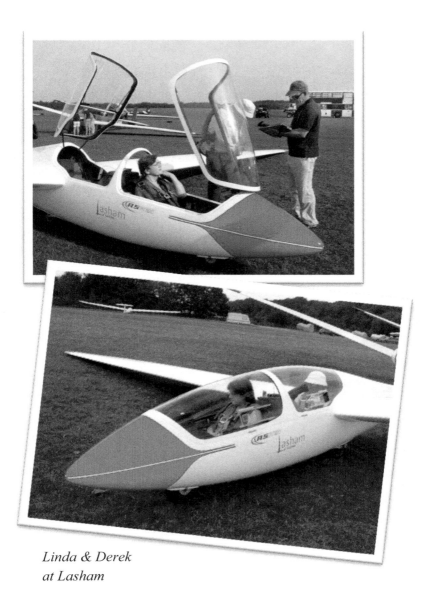

*Linda & Derek
at Lasham*

CHAPTER 8

GET 'EM OUT BY FRIDAY

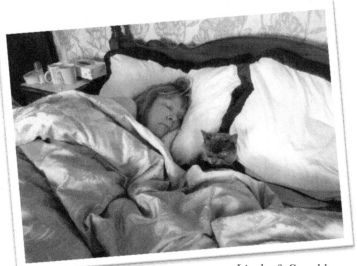

*Linda & Sparkle
cuddling at Dwygyfylchi*

Back in Chipperfield there was more work to do, on cars, by necessity, and for dogs, always the more rewarding. We were also thinking of ways to help the boys and in early 2013 we looked into the possibility of buying Linda's council house, in which she had lived for 25 years, improving it beyond measure from the condition in which she and John took it over when Alex was very small and Dan was due. It was therefore the only home they'd known and I rang the council to tell them the position and was advised to put in an application. Ultimately it was rejected because it was not Linda's 'principal home', even though I'd told them where she was living and why. No amount of discussion would change their minds, and the woman I'd spoken to initially never figured in subsequent negotiations, despite my requests that she be included.

We also asked if the boys could take on the tenancy and rent the house themselves but this idea was also rejected, so Linda was evicted and so were the boys. The council cited the need to house families in the area, and never replied to my question regarding the single man who lived in the adjoining three-bedroom house, apparently that was ok, but they had to throw two young men out of an identical house which had been their only home.

I also raised the issue that had been brought up by then-chancellor George Osborne about possible cuts being made for high earners living in council houses. A BBC article at the time states 'Issues that he did highlight as possible areas for savings were the payment of housing benefit to people aged under 25 and also people living in council houses while earning more than £65,000 per year' and this was in 2013. FYI, council houses are supposed to be 'affordable homes for those of modest means', and no, the boys did not earn that much money, nowhere near, but they were still thrown out of their home.

Chapter 9

You Made Me
A Nervous Wreck

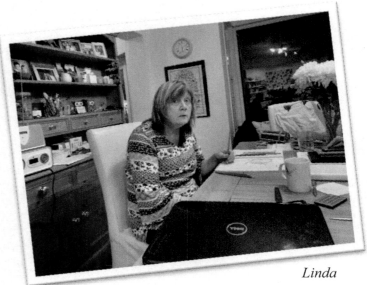

Linda
"in the office"

In the autumn we returned to stay for a little while at Conwy Marina, but were able to dismiss the idea of living there. It was too near the western end of the Conwy River tunnel, which carries the North Wales Expressway/A55, and it was simply too noisy for us. Something else to take into consideration when choosing suitable accommodation was whether it had a bathroom, by which I mean a room with a bath, not just a shower, (that would be a shower room). Plenty of places claim to have a bathroom, but they actually have a shower room.

Why does this matter? Because I need to shower Linda while she's sitting down, on a bath board, supported on a bath, with a handheld/portable shower head, (I often do this whilst singing 'Car wash' by Rose Royce) and this can be difficult to track down. Sometimes we've had to struggle in a tiny shower cubicle together, and as someone who can't stand showers anyway, it makes things ten times worse. These will normally have a fixed shower head so basically, we both just get wet, any soap or shampoo gets rinsed away almost immediately and we wish we hadn't bothered. Wet rooms? Don't start me on wet rooms, oh alright then, what a waste of space. The bather gets wet, and so does the carer, and so do the towels, the toilet paper and anything else in the line of fire, worst things since decking, don't start me on decking...

Problems were also brewing at 'Rosemary', which is accessed from the road along a 200ft long sloping drive. The drive had been there ever since the bungalow was built in the mid 30's, long before the neighbouring bungalow, which for some strange reason assumed ownership of it, even though we had legal rights to use it.

Despite Linda's condition, the owners decided to dig up the drive to 'repair' it, completely against my wishes, even though it was perfectly serviceable. So, we had to rely on our dear Welsh neighbour to retain access to our home during this time. He had very kindly allowed my father to walk across his garden to get to Chipperfield Common some years before, and at this time he allowed me to park my car at his house so that we wouldn't be blocked in.

One evening I took Linda to see a film at Sarratt village hall, the next village along, and we had to clamber through the hedge, past the vegetable plots and around the pitch-dark garden to 'defy the ban'.

These incidents might not have made Linda's condition worse, but they certainly weren't helping, and early in 2014 worse was to come. The neighbours tried to stop me working on cars at home, even though I'd only worked on 30 cars during the whole year, and the council officer I originally spoke to had said it was perfectly ok to do so.

The neighbour in question had over the years progressively hampered our access along the driveway and this was clearly another knee-jerk reaction to my endeavours to keep the drive clear for access. I'd been working on cars for nearly seven years without complaint, but all of a sudden it was an issue.

We'd already decided to move right away. If we'd stayed in the area, it would probably have been in or near Tring, but though there are plenty of reservoirs in Tring there aren't any mountains, and it'll be a long time before Tring has any beaches.

We sold the house and decided to move out on the 5th June, with my friend Martin supervising the removal company on the next day to ensure that everything was rounded up and headed north without interruption from the neighbours. It had taken a long time to pack, with youngest son Danny helping to get things down from the loft and Julia coming over from Willesden to help. She also did a lot to interpret and relay Linda's feelings and wishes to myself. Julia carefully wrapped numerous delicate items in particular and we were very grateful for her help.

So, on Thursday June 5th we set off - Linda, Lucy and me. Apart from getting stuck in a hold up near Stoke on the M5, we got to Llandudno Junction in the early evening and called the estate agent who was handling the rental property we'd taken on for six months while we looked for somewhere permanent.

CHAPTER 10

AIN'T NO SUNSHINE

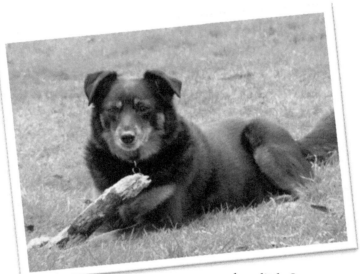

...dear little Lucy xx

W e'd not seen it before we arrived, but Ken, from 'Tan yr Allt', had checked it over for us, along with some other properties, and thought it would be suitable. It was a modern link detached, with nice neighbours who made tea for the removal men who'd travelled all the way from Amersham.

We couldn't stay there the first night so Ken and Sue put us up at their house and we moved in properly the next day. It was a tight squeeze but anything we didn't need immediately was stacked in the hall, and the garage, and in the living room, and the spare bedroom. You get the picture.

The big worry now was Lucy. I had tried to get her teeth cleaned the previous autumn but, as she was 11 and needed a general anaesthetic, the vet carried out blood tests and found that her liver function was poor and that she wouldn't cope. So, from then on we knew her days were numbered, but had no idea how long they would be.

The 'new' vet we went to in Llandudno saw my Tiggywinkles (Wildlife hospital near Aylesbury) Polo shirt and it turned out she was from Aylesbury and had worked at Tiggys some years before, whereas I had volunteered there in 2002/3. She treated Lucy over the next few weeks and I kept her on the special hepatic diet, which she really didn't like, but as usual I was stuck in that cleft stick of wanting her to live forever and wanting the best quality of life for her as well. She was still as lively as ever, and was still racing up and down the stairs regularly and walking normally but one evening a lot of fluid had to be drawn off her tummy. She seemed much better and didn't appear to be suffering at all.

The next day we all drove to the airfield near Denbigh to meet Derek, who was flying up from Hampshire in a powered glider. It was July 25th, a very hot day, and after a few hours he set off back home in the early evening and we drove back to the house.

That evening we were expecting Danny and his girlfriend Lois to bring her family dog Bobby for us to look after. When they arrived, I went out to the car and when Danny and I hugged, he noticed that the back of my shirt was wet from where I'd been sitting cuddling Lucy moments before. That was it, we found her trying to hide under a bush in the back garden and I knew then that she'd had enough and called the vet to the house. She offered to give more treatment but I knew it would only prolong the inevitable and didn't want her to suffer at all so as we all sat with her, all except Bobby, we said our goodbyes to my dear little Lucy.

She'd been found dumped as a puppy at Luton airport, in carpark C, hence her name, and she'd come to me when she was only about 8 or 9 months old. She was only 12.

Chapter 11

Let's Get Married

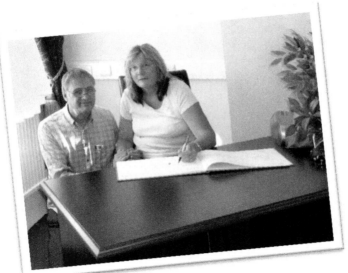

Our glitzy "High Society Wedding"

L osing Lucy was something I was ready for, even though I didn't know when it might be, so that helped take the sting out of the situation to some extent. We also had little Bobby to help take our minds off things for a couple of weeks. Bobbie was a Westie with a penchant for cucumber and a habit of barking wildly whenever the bell rang to announce that a new order was ready at the cafe in Conwy's Castle Street.

Two more significant events happened while we were living in Victoria drive, the first was when Linda and I paid a visit to Llandudno town hall and were married on September 18th. We'd notified them in advance of course but had no witnesses or friends to help us, but as they had promised, the town hall staff found us two witnesses. Whereas Linda used to live in Welwyn Garden City and work in Hatfield, it turned out that one of the witnesses, who was working on a theatre production in the town hall, used to live in Hatfield and work in Welwyn Garden City. Luckily the

Paparazzi didn't get wind of the event so everything passed off quietly just as we wished.

The next big event was our trip to Ireland in late September, part-modest honeymoon and part-mission to repatriate Billie, who'd been staying with a lovely couple in County Galway for the summer. We were now living less than an hour away from Holyhead so we took the opportunity to cross the Irish sea on the 'Jonathan Swift' ferry and head west for the town of Portumna. This was a welcome break in what was really an Indian summer, complete with flocks of swallows massing on the phone lines in the fields adjacent to Karen and John's house, and several sightseeing trips. We also got to finally see Galway Bay and the city itself in glorious weather.

On our return we had to focus on choosing a 'new' house, and among the contenders were a former Franciscan Friary in

Penmaenmawr, which sadly would have needed too much work to adapt to our needs, and a third of a big house at the top of the Sychnant pass above Conwy, complete with four acres of land. This would have been ideal as I've always wanted an animal sanctuary, and even if I couldn't manage it myself it would have been lovely to enable it and to see it filled with rescued animals. I had to agree with Linda though that the house itself wasn't ideal for us, and it was a bit remote, so attention turned to the former 'Gordon Villa' in Glan Conwy.

When I'd first seen it on the adverts, I'd thought it was too good to be true. When we turned up to look at it, I realised that actually, it was true. Built in 1890 and set at right angles to the road so that the occupant, who also owned ships, could see them sailing up the river Conwy into the port (sadly no longer there) in the village. Apparently, it was named Gordon villa after General Gordon of Khartoum as patriotic fervour was all the rage at the time, we know it as Number 18.

It's been extended a couple of times, the first by the addition of a cottage at the end nearest to the road, probably not long after the main house was built. This was ideal as we needed somewhere to let out for income and Fiona the vet, who lived just up the road, happened to find us the ideal candidate. Tanja was a German vet nurse who applied to join Fiona's surgery and needed local accommodation. She got the job and she got our cottage and boy were we glad. She turned out to be the perfect tenant and has become a good friend into the bargain. When she left two years ago, it was to move into her own place in the village and before she went, she found us more perfect tenants for the cottage; Andrew, Lorraine and their lovely little dog Harry, vielen danke Tanja!

On our previous visits we'd already discovered the local Stroke Group and the

North Wales Brain Injury Service (NWBIS), both at Colwyn Bay, and the group became a weekly appointment that we rarely missed. The Stroke Association had stopped funding this group some time previously but the ladies who ran it carried on doing so on a purely voluntary basis and regularly had 15-20 patients on every Wednesday afternoon. I got Linda there for 2pm and went off to walk Billie, who had now come to live with us, at Eirias park, just over the road, or by the river at Llanddulas, on the way to Abergele. Linda enjoyed many different activities there and on occasion there were musical events and outings too. Sadly the group folded at the start of lockdown and is no longer in existence.

As early as July 24th we received a visit from Julie, an Occupational Therapist working for NWBIS, who arranged for a referral to the Occupational Therapy workshop at the Bryn y Neuadd Hospital in Llanfairfechan. We also started getting used to official letters printed in Welsh and English, and recognising the various accents we were hearing. A traditional Welsh accent is really what spoken English sounds like in the South and Mid Wales, while English spoken in North Wales sounds more like Northern English, but the speakers are far more likely to be bi-lingual and to speak Welsh as their first choice. In my experience they will always politely switch if English-only speakers are present however.

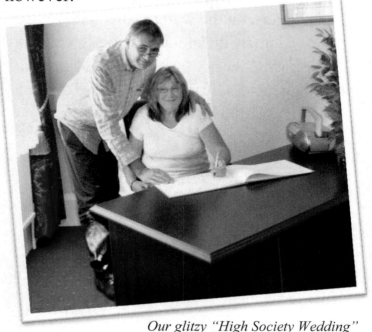

Our glitzy "High Society Wedding"

CHAPTER 12

A DESIGN FOR LIFE

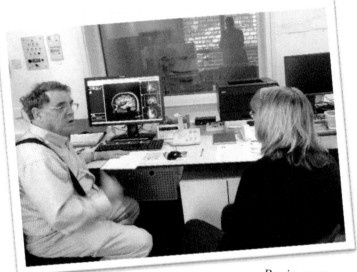

*Brain scan
at Bangor University*

A lthough the rental house served its purpose it was very cramped and cluttered and I will always associate it as well with Lucy's passing, so we were very pleased to eventually settle on the purchase of number 18 and we finally moved in, as far as I can remember, on Tuesday the 14th October, the removal team being cheerfully and expertly led by Phil, himself a resident of Glan Conwy.

As well as quickly adapting to our new home we were more than happy to get used to another novel situation, lovely neighbours. On both sides we were delighted to find wonderful people who made us feel welcome and were to prove immensely helpful and kind to us over the years. Billie settled in well and though we had a garden the presence of the adjacent 'Acre field' has been another bonus as we can access it straight from our garden and dogs can socialise together as they need to, and enjoy doing so.

The house did need some urgent modifications however. The first was to fit an extra handrail to the staircase as there was only one on the left side going up, the banister rail, but none on the other side, which was the wall, and what was the wall largely made of ? Lath and plaster that's what, which is not terribly good at load bearing. In one location I had to modify the wall to make it strong enough to fit the necessary bracket and so far, it's worked and Linda has something to hold on to on either side. In some situations she's had to come down stairs backwards so she's been able to keep hold of the only rail.

The other place that needed prompt attention was the bathroom, it was very pretty and all that, with a free-standing bath, a separate shower cubicle and two washbasins, but completely impractical for us. It was soon dismantled and remodelled with a large standard bath with a shower over and one basin, sorted.

Linda was soon attending the OT workshop at Llanfairfechan, a wonderful facility dedicated mainly to woodworking, and fully equipped and adapted to cater for people with various disabilities. The team of three who ran the workshop were lovely to deal with and Linda very much enjoyed her two separate stints there, with the added bonus for both of us being that transport was laid on for her so I could stay usefully occupied at home whilst it was extra independence for her.

Her efforts at the workshop produced a sturdy garden bench, a bird feeder, a planter and a trug, all still gainfully employed. There were two stints because each is for a fixed term but luckily another vacancy occurred soon after the first one ended. Serious efforts were also made to address the problems with spasticity in Linda's right hand, with regular visits to Glan Clwyd and Colwyn Bay physiotherapy departments, with various splint devices specially made for her.

Our GP also agreed to a referral to neurology for assessment for botox injections and in the meantime, he prescribed baclofen although sadly this didn't seem to help at all.

We also dealt with the Royal Alexandra Hospital in Rhyl who created a foot splint to try to help her with the right foot which was twisted to one side and 'dropped', causing problems with walking. All this happened within a few months of our arrival and we felt so grateful for all the assistance we'd experienced in such a short space of time, quite a novelty after the relative lack of attention we received in Hertfordshire.

As well as the splints, which are updated at regular intervals, we were supplied with specially made shoes which are also updated when necessary. In Hertfordshire we had to source and pay for our own shoes from a gentleman in Hatfield but they were not as appropriate for Linda's needs as the ones we have now. We had a brief flirtation with the FFIT gym at Llandudno Junction but didn't get on with the different types of equipment and gave it up as a bad job. We really needed a dedicated trainer to help us but none was available.

Various meetings at North Wales Brain Injury Service however had thrown up the possibility of assessment and treatment at Bangor University as I mentioned earlier, specifically the 'Wolfson Centre for Clinical and Cognitive Neuroscience' at the School of Psychology based in the Brigantia Building.

We attended several times for Linda to undergo tests, the main diagnostic session taking place on Thursday the 30th April 2015 involving an extremely detailed MRI scan conducted by American Professor Bob Rafal. Billie came with us on all of these visits and waited patiently for Mum to have her tests, copies of which we were given on DVD. This MRI was of a much higher resolution than the normal NHS scans and the upshot was that they were amazed at the amount of movement, speech and understanding Linda had retained after such widespread brain damage.

They were unable to assist Linda in more practical ways but all of them, particularly Becca Henderson, were very kind and helpful and we are still in touch with Dr. Giovanni D'Avossa, who we see from time to time at NWBIS. Shortly before lockdown he approved our acceptance on an advanced Aphasia treatment programme at the National Hospital for Neurology and Neurosurgery at University college London which sadly, we have been unable to attend so far due to the pandemic.

Did we discover any more advantages of living in Wales? Apart from being a beautiful country with a fascinating history, the oldest living language in Europe and what has been voted the coolest flag in the world, we found we would receive free prescriptions as a matter of national policy and free parking at all NHS hospitals. Ok, you've talked us into it.

Oh, as Columbo would say, 'one more thing', we were issued with a HYNT card. This is issued by the Arts council of Wales and improves access to theatre and music venues for disabled people and their carers. In effect it halves the cost of admission for the customer and their carer and has helped us to see such great acts at Venue Cymru in Llandudno as Joe Brown, Jasper Carrott, Milton Jones, Al Murray, KT Tunstall, Amy MacDonald, Level 42, James, The Coral, Manic Street Preachers, and my guitar hero Nils Lofgren, as well as a recording of 'I'm sorry I haven't a clue'. There are other benefits of the scheme and yet again it seems to be exclusively Welsh, diolch yn fawr Cymru!

It was at the end of 2014 that Tanja moved into our attached annexe with her black cat Loki and it was in mid-2015 that we 'adopted' a homeless cat that had taken to sleeping in our shed, our builder Barry who was doing various jobs around the house got him to overcome his fear and start to come into the house more, (Barry having four cats himself he was more in tune with them), and I decided to call him Frankie. He and Billie got on fine although he and Loki didn't get on quite as well.

In May that year we drove to Loughborough to collect my sister Anna and then we carried on to Norfolk to attend the celebration of the 75th anniversary of the founding of the Czech squadrons in the RAF during WW2. Dad had been a wireless operator in 311 squadron and flew Wellington bombers from East Wretham during 1940 and 1941 and the occasion was marked by an exhibition at the local church. One of the most poignant sights was the old tree on the edge of the airfield where the Czech aircrew would meet to pray before their missions. Dad made 39 operational flights from East Wretham and Honington totalling nearly 200 hours over occupied Europe. While there we also visited the aviation museum at the airport at Norwich, the city where Dad met my Mum at Christmas time 1940.

On May 25th Linda, Billie and I drove to Liverpool to see the '3 Queens', the largest of the Cunard ships, Victoria, Elizabeth and Mary 2, all together in the Mersey to celebrate 175 years of the Cunard line. Quite a sight, and a great deal of flag waving, though sad to say two of the ships were built in Italy and the other was built in France. Oh, and they're all registered in Bermuda. At least the Red Arrows overhead were built in Britain.

About one month later we all drove down to Pembrokeshire to meet Linda's brother Gary as he finished his charity walk along the coastal path. We stayed near Talbenny airfield and found some more buildings that had survived since Dad's time on Coastal Command, along with pictures of other

Czech airmen. On the way back we stopped to meet my friends Kathy and Ben at Newport, near Fishguard, Ben's father had also been in the RAF, he was a Polish Spitfire pilot during WW2.

In August we went to Rhyl to see the air show, the star of which was definitely the Vulcan bomber. It's huge, it's fast, and it's incredibly manoeuvrable, an awesome machine. The town was packed but we found a great place to watch from near the boating lake and model railway and I managed to get some good pictures of the Vulcan.

It turned out to be quite an eventful year because our next trip was to my beloved Isle of Man, taking in the Manx car rally and catching up with old friends. Barry the builder stayed in the house to finish off some work he'd been doing and we left Billie and Frankie in his care for the week.

The next year however started with a bang, literally. Just back from the Cross Keys on a dark, damp Sunday evening (and no, I hadn't drunk too much) I decided to take a look at an area of decking at the top of the garden. I'm sure it must have seemed like a good idea at the time, but turning to go back inside I soon realised that I'd slipped and instantly gone from vertical to horizontal. Fortunately however my fall was stopped by the back of my head. As the lights dimmed and almost immediately switched back on again, I realised I was still conscious, losing blood, and in trouble. I called out for help once before realising it was a waste of time and energy and managed to grope my way back into the kitchen to present the new version of myself to a shocked Linda and Billie.

I think they preferred the previous version and I must say I did as well, but the first worry was how I could care for Linda and Billie in this condition. I must have had to call for the ambulance myself and when the crew arrived, they said something along the lines of 'WE REALLY THINK YOU

SHOULD GO TO HOSPITAL', to which I said 'Who's going to look after my disabled wife and fifteen-year-old dog? I think they must have gone next door and asked Alan and Yvonne to pop round and they were marvellous. Alan actually followed the ambulance to Glan Clwyd hospital and Yvonne stayed to make sure Linda and Billie were ok, although I think I must have got Billie's food ready before we went.

I was a long time waiting in the ambulance but was eventually admitted and Alan stayed with me the whole night until I could be treated, the wait being used to conduct observations to ensure I didn't need anything more than stitches. These were duly administered without anaesthetic at about 5am while Alan watched on. I must say he didn't look as if he wanted to swap places. He then drove us home and can't have got much sleep as he had to work that day. What a wonderful gesture that was, and so appreciated. I had always dreaded something happening to put me out of action and leaving Linda without assistance but these wonderful neighbours did all they could to help out and it wasn't the last occasion we've had cause to be grateful to them.

I'd always been wary of the decking and knew how slippery and out of bounds it was when wet, which let's face it, is quite often. Just how slippery and indeed deadly it could be convinced me it had to go and the largest area of it has now been replaced with paving. The small areas that remain will be covered with anti-slip material and in the meantime, I'm giving them a very wide berth. Another neighbour also slipped on his decking about a year ago, seriously injuring his back, last time I checked he was still waiting for an operation. Wet rooms, decking and food served on wooden boards can all join each other in room 101 as far as I'm concerned - modern fads that are definitely more trouble than they're worth.

In July we boarded the MV Balmoral at Llandudno Pier and set off for a trip around Anglesey. The open water was pretty rough though and it wasn't all that easy to move around inside the ship so were pleased to start the last leg of the journey by entering the sheltered waters of the Menai strait at Caernarfon. There was much more to see along the banks of the strait and whilst we'd driven over them many times, it was fascinating to pass under the wonderful bridges built by Telford and Stephenson nearly two centuries before.

We also went on a coach tour of the quarries at Penmaenmawr mountain one very hot evening. These had provided enormous amounts of granite and other materials over the years, reducing the mountain, which had once risen almost vertically to 1600 feet, to about 1000 feet.

The views from the top were still breathtaking though, across Anglesey and the coast of North Wales, and it was good to get a close-up view of one of our favourite local landmarks, the quarry clock high up on the hillside which can be seen from just about anywhere in the town.

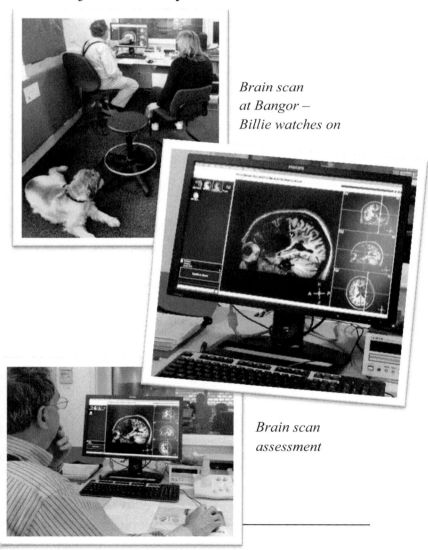

*Brain scan
at Bangor –
Billie watches on*

*Brain scan
assessment*

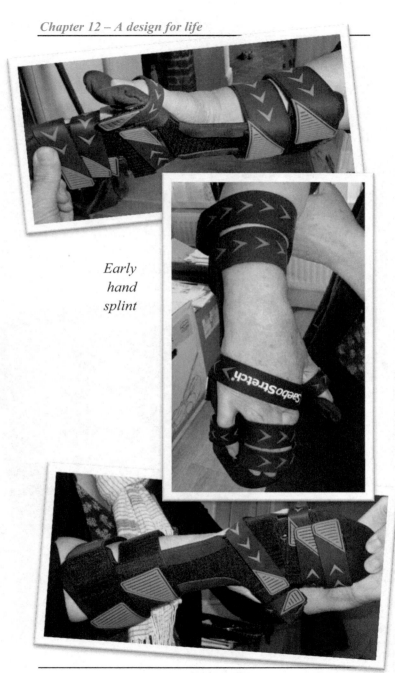

*Early
hand
splint*

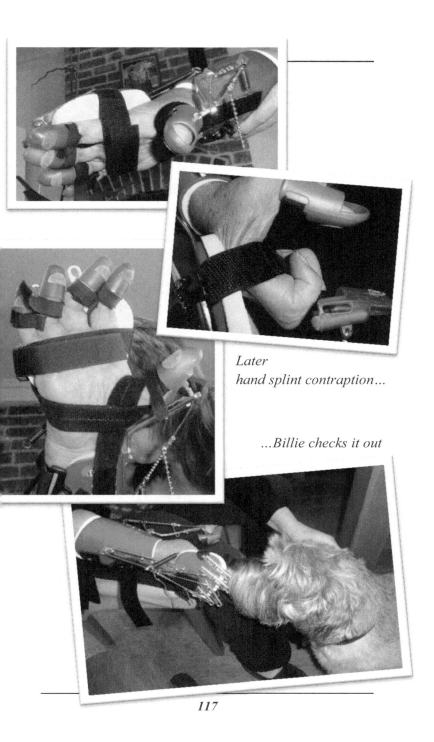

*Later
hand splint contraption...*

...Billie checks it out

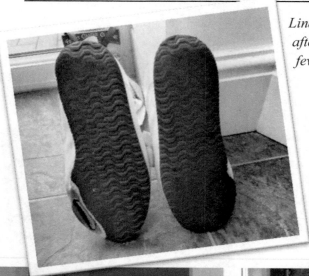

*Linda's shoes
after a
few weeks wear*

*Linda's
bench*

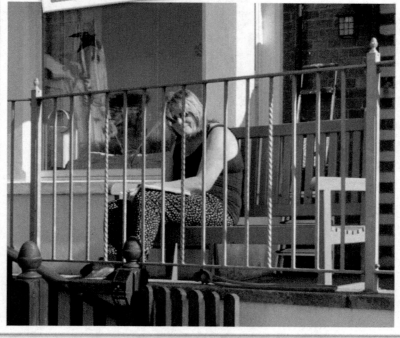

Rhyl – Linda at the
Miniature Railway

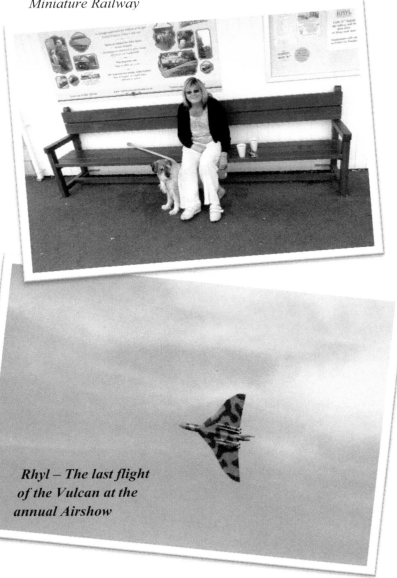

Rhyl – The last flight
of the Vulcan at the
annual Airshow

CHAPTER 13

DEEPLY DIPPY

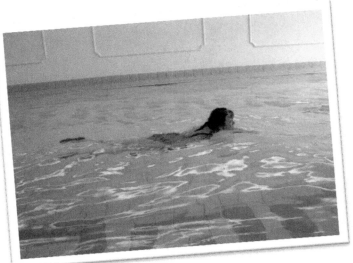

*Swimming
at Mint Imperial*

All this time of course Linda was carrying on with the stroke group and the OT workshop, but another beneficial activity was on the horizon - swimming. We had been attending the nearby Leonard Cheshire home at Colwyn Heights for hydrotherapy for some time but Linda wanted to swim properly again so I started looking around for a suitable venue. She used to swim regularly but hadn't been able to since the stroke, indeed the likelihood of doing so hadn't even cropped up as there were more pressing matters to cope with. It didn't help that I can't swim so couldn't take her myself, because she still needs someone with her in the water. When the idea of her actually swimming again took hold, I started looking for places where someone was available to teach/safeguard her and I found that the Imperial Hotel in Llandudno had a gym and swimming pool in the basement. It's called 'Mint Imperial', see what they did there?

There was a teacher available as well although the changing room wasn't suitable for her so we used a spare room for the few occasions we were there. I say a few because the teacher seemed to spend most of her time in Dorset, and the pool wasn't all that big either, so after a few sessions I switched the venue to Rhydal Penrhos school in Colwyn Bay.

The pool there is much bigger and there was a teacher available full time as well, and we used this arrangement for a couple of years. I would help Linda get down the steps into the water and Theresa would take over. Of course, it took a while before Linda got used to swimming again at all and indeed to swimming with only one arm, we thought she might go round in circles at first but I'm glad to say she proved us all wrong and went up and down as straight as a Troy Deeney penalty. She did use a float on her right arm most of the time but even managed without that eventually and was soon able to be escorted up and down the pool and also to do exercises in the water on her own.

I would then help her out of the water and back to the changing room as she is not all that steady on her feet, especially on the slippery walkway around the edge.

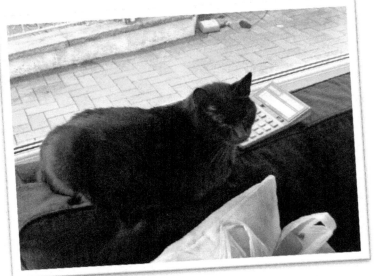

Frankie,
doing the accounts

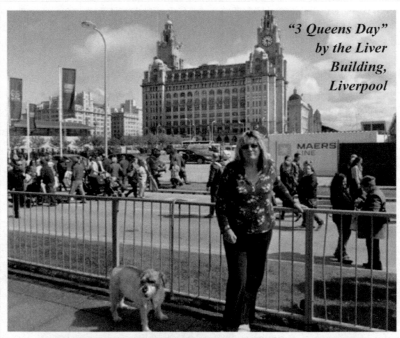

"3 Queens Day" by the Liver Building, Liverpool

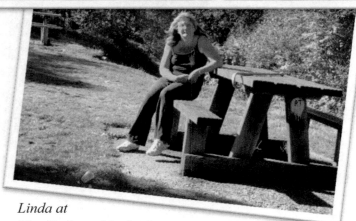

Linda at Llyn Padarn, Llanberis

CHAPTER 14

I DON'T
WANNA TALK ABOUT IT

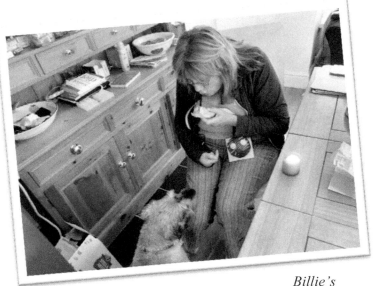

*Billie's
birthday*

In the autumn of 2016, we travelled to the Lake district for a few days and Billie came too of course. Sadly, we couldn't see as much of the scenery as we'd have liked for obvious reasons, except from the car.

2017 was approaching and what a challenge it turned out to be. We were visited in April by Maria Harvey from the 'Electronic Assistive Technology Service' based in Cardiff, so that Linda could be assessed for any available help with her communication requirements. I had hoped that something like the system that Stephen Hawking used could be employed but this requires that the user can picture and spell the words they want to use in their mind and sadly Linda is unable to do so. Maria did however supply us with an iPad with a programme called 'Proloquo2go' installed, and this was loaded with phrases and photos that Linda could use to convey information to other people. Tanja took pictures of our pub regulars, and we added family pics and of course, pictures of our associated dogs and cats and it has proved useful to her.

But it was at the beginning of June that my biggest worry manifested itself again, with the onset of illness and my inability to care for Linda and Billie.

On Sunday 4th June I felt 'a bit ropey' in the evening and when Monday morning arrived, I was feeling very ill indeed. I don't normally get headaches but this was a cracker, along with other symptoms. Come evening time Billie, who'd been fading in recent days, was no longer able to climb the stairs to our room where she always slept. I felt so awful I remember saying that there was no chance I'd have the strength to carry her up but she became so distressed I had to force myself to pick her up and take her up to our bedroom.

The next day I finally called the surgery and they told me to call an ambulance. The crew checked me over and came to the conclusion that they didn't know what was

wrong with me, which wasn't really what I
wanted to hear, especially as, no word of a
lie, if I'd had a gun handy I'm pretty sure
I'd have used it (on me, not the ambulance
crew). I'd never felt so ill. Off they went
leaving me even more concerned and later
on Tanja had a chat with my neighbour Dan
to tell him how worried she was. As far as I
remember, because she was working that
evening, he persuaded me to get in his car
and took me to Glan Clwyd hospital. I took
some convincing because I was so worried
about Linda and Billie but it was obviously
the right thing to do. I remember looking at
the speedo in Dan's Volvo as we drove
through Llanddulas on the A55 at xxxmph
and we were soon in A&E reception and
not so soon being 'interviewed' by a
particularly cynical doctor who tried to trip
me up on details of my story. I pointed out
that I was feeling very ill indeed and
certainly not up for a contest in semantics
and he cleared me for triage, which only
happened after another couple of hours

lying on a bench in the waiting room while Tuesday became Wednesday.

I'll draw a veil over my experiences in the next two weeks though. I was worried how Linda would cope and can remember asking about social services getting in touch, I knew that Tanja would be doing her best to help though and was able to accept that there was nothing more I could do at the time. Someone must have brought my laptop and phone and I remember telling people on Facebook where I was and eldest son Alex must have come up to stay with his Mum quite early on. I think he went back on the Sunday, 11th June, and as bad luck would have it, that was when Billie took a real turn for the worse.

Linda must have managed to get down to Alan and Yvonne's house next door. It's a bit awkward for her because there are some narrow steps involved, but they both came round to help her and Alan rang me to say he'd take Billie to the vets. I thanked him but was pretty sure what the outcome would be and didn't want her to be upset any more than necessary so asked him to get the vet to come to the house and to call me when they arrived. The vet came on the phone and we agreed that Billie should be helped on her way to the Rainbow bridge and asked for the phone to be put to Billie's ear.

When I spoke to her to tell her that all was going to be well and all the dogs she knew that she was going to see again she barked and everyone in the room said she knew it was me so that was some small comfort. She was 16 years old and had done really well and been a wonderful companion for us. It was such a shame too that Linda was alone with her that night but so reassuring to know that our neighbours would be so kind and thoughtful.

Danny came up to stay the next week, my brother came up from Hertfordshire and collected my sister from Leicestershire on the way and visited me during the week. I remember with horror seeing the tv pictures of the Grenfell tower fire in the early hours of Wednesday 14th June. Linda was being brought to see me of course and our friend Sara from the village also came and I can only assume that by now Linda was being supported as much as she needed to be.

I think it was the next Monday or Tuesday that I was allowed to go home and was very pleased that Tanja came to collect me. The weather had been unbearably hot for the duration and I was so pleased to get back to some sort of normality. Yet again we were so grateful to Glan Clwyd hospital and the power of antibiotics. At first, they'd thought I might have meningitis, hence two lumbar punctures, but it was actually pneumonia. Someone subsequently said "oh, it's 'cos of your age"(65), I told them I'd also had pneumonia when I was 8.

By early July we were more-or-less back to whatever normal is. Linda going swimming, having botox at Caernarfon etc and we made a snap decision to get away for a few days to Aberystwyth, a place I remember fondly as the first where a complete stranger called me 'bach', a Welsh term of endearment. While there we took a ride on the funicular cliff railway, visited the camera obscura, and took a lovely trip on the Vale of Rheidol steam railway to Devil's Bridge, whilst on the way back home we looked in at the Dyfi Osprey Centre just south of Machynlleth.

In August Linda started attending the 'She shed', an offshoot of the Men's shed, at Colwyn Bay. Essentially this is a woodworking facility that includes tea, conversation and lots of sawdust and we attended a few times but Linda didn't really take to it. Well worth a try though.

At the end of the month, I also took Linda to see a homoeopath at Colwyn Bay but the treatment produced no results at all. I'll never stop looking for ways to improve her condition though.

In early October my friend Derek travelled all the way from Hertfordshire to Aboyne airfield near Aberdeen to indulge his passion for gliding, and on the way, he collected us and took us as far as Falkirk to enable me to collect a 'new' car. It seemed like a good idea at the time. At Falkirk we saw the beautiful Kelpies, the largest equine statues in the world, and the incredible Falkirk wheel, the world's first and only rotating boat lift. Falkirk, world leading or what?

We then stayed for a couple of days near Glasgow, one of my favourite places, and was pleased that Linda also enjoyed the Kelvingrove museum and the Riverside Museum on the Clyde as well as a drive along the west bank of Loch Lomond.

November saw us heading south instead, a four-hour drive through the heart of Wales and stunning scenery brought us to the capital, Cardiff. We were attending the first stroke assembly for patients and carers in Wales, held at the Copthorne hotel, a mile or two west of the city centre. I guess we were hoping to learn of some new research or treatment that could help Linda but though the lectures and personal testimonies of stroke survivors proved interesting, we sadly heard nothing that would help us in our particular situation. The few days in Cardiff were very enjoyable though, it's a wonderful city.

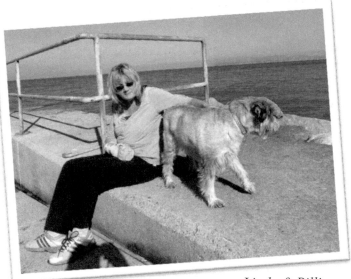

Linda & Billie
at Penmaenmawr

CHAPTER 15

SYNCHRONICITY

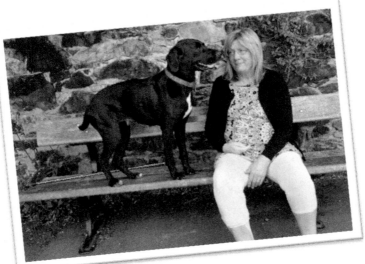

Linda & Senna at Marine Walk,
Conwy – my favourite picture

The end of 2017 was also significant for a wonderful reason. I was talking with a friend in the Cross Keys on Christmas eve and he asked when we were getting another dog. "When we make the back garden more secure" I told him. "What dog will you get?" he asked. "Any dog that needs a home" I said. "Where will you get the dog from?" he asked. "I'm sure a dog will find us" I replied. For this story to make full sense you'll need to know that when (with my parents) we had two rescued staffie crosses, I called the first one Pepsi, and the second one Niki, after Niki Lauda.

So, on the morning of Christmas day, Dave from the pub rang me and told me that his brother-in-law was visiting from Nantwich with his dog and that he couldn't look after her properly as his wife and children had left him and he was working full time. Dave apparently had no idea that this situation would arise and having persuaded the brother-in-law to rehome the dog he realised that there were two options. One was the local RSPCA centre at Bryn y Maen, and the other was me. He said that she was a four-and-a-half-year-old Labrador/Pointer Cross. Her name? Senna. (If any young people are reading this, please find an older person and ask them who Ayrton Senna was).

Well, I didn't really need to even see her, it was obvious she was meant for us and we took her on immediately, she is an absolute delight and we both adore her.

2018 saw another new arrival, Linda's first granddaughter, Riley, was born to Danny and Lois in St.Albans on April 18th and as soon as we could, we went down south to see her.

August was noticeable for sad and happy reasons. My dear friend Margy Bruin passed away having suffered from Parkinsons for several years, but at least she had the dedicated support of her older sister Judi, who had an extension built on to her house so that she could look after her.

I went down on my own to her funeral in Amersham on what must have been the hottest day of the year, another reminder of what a good decision it was to move to a more even climate. It was Margy who looked after Lucy on the day of Linda's stroke and was the most wonderful person.

Later in the month though saw our return to the Isle of Man after a three-year absence, this time to see the Manx Grand Prix and Classic TT and to introduce Senna to the Island. We booked to stay with a family in Douglas who had their own dog and were all set to leave on Tuesday the 21st. On Monday evening Senna started coughing, so badly that I had to take her to the vet. Diagnosis? Kennel cough. Result? Senna had to stay behind, lest she passed it to our host's dog. Luckily the vet herself offered to care for Senna for the next fortnight, and during that time she also managed to spay her.

When Senna arrived that Christmas morning she was in rather poor condition. She had mange and kept having phantom pregnancies. The mange was quickly dispatched but the phantoms kept happening. Her stay at the vets then was an ideal opportunity to keep tabs on her and choose the right time to operate and we were sent video updates as well so we knew she was getting the best of care. Hopefully she'll be with us the next time we board the Manx ferry. As usual our time in the Island was a delight. The family we stayed with was lovely, and the only practical problem Linda had was getting on and off the electric tram that took us to the summit of Snaefell.

Linda had had to stop attending the workshop at Llanfairfechan sometime before but was now trying art therapy, with sessions at Llandudno and Abergele, but along with the stroke group itself, these have stopped due to Covid. She enjoyed these activities and being with other people and being independent for a while but she has obviously been badly affected psychologically as well as physically by the stroke, and at times she's had problems with alcohol, which is hardly surprising, but has caused some issues that had to be addressed. We both also had other medical conditions that needed regular treatment and life has sometimes been difficult but never more so than when communication has been the stumbling block. The frustrations Linda feels are almost tangible at times and it's heart-breaking to see this wonderful person struggling to make herself understood so very often.

She was always quiet and undemonstrative, delightfully easy to talk to, with no pretensions or dramatics, and now I can't even remember the sound of her voice, I'd love to hear it again. All I can do most of the time is try to take her out as much as possible to enjoy our surroundings and more far-flung places as well. In February 2019 this meant a trip to Bedford for the marriage of Alex and Samantha. We stayed at the wedding venue on the banks of the river Ouse. It's a very dog-friendly place and Senna came along too of course.

Very sadly though we lost Frankie, probably to a road accident, when we got back. We had always thought he was sufficiently street wise to keep out of trouble on the road outside but he'd been living rough before we took him in and had continued to roam. We'd installed a cat flap for him and he'd got used to using it, but one morning poor Tanja found him dead outside her cottage. We'll never be completely sure what happened but the most likely explanation is that he was hit a glancing blow from a passing car. He and Senna got on fine, as he had with Billie, and it was quite a shock for us all.

In June there was an exhibition of work from the art groups, this took place at Porth Eirias in Colwyn Bay and all the contributors were stroke survivors including Linda of course. Also in the summer, youngest son Danny, who had been having personal problems, came to stay with us for a few months and as he is a former county springboard diver for Hertfordshire you won't be surprised to hear that he can swim and was able to take his Mum to the pool at Llandudno a few times. This was easier for Linda to access than the other pools she'd used as she could walk down a gentle slope at one side into deeper water.

This all went by the board again when Covid struck the next year but hopefully we'll restart these sessions again for her as soon as we can. Yet again, the end of the year saw us taking to the road again, first of all to celebrate Tanja's birthday in July by crossing the famous Pontcysyllte aqueduct near Llangollen, where the Llangollen canal passes over the river Dee. It's the highest aqueduct in the world and the longest in Great Britain and passing along it high over the Dee valley in a narrow boat is quite an experience.

We also set off to the North East to stay at first in Seahouses, stepping off point for the Farne Islands, and as well as a boat trip to see the seabirds that nest there in the summer, we travelled up the coast and crossed the causeway to Lindisfarne. I've always loved the band named after the island but sadly the place itself was packed with people the day we went and far too busy for us to be able to take our time to enjoy the experience. This actually worked in our favour though because we decided to head north up the coast to Berwick and we both fell head over heels with the place.

From the first view of the beautiful bridge that carries traffic over the river Tweed to the wonderful early evening boat trip we took to see dolphins leaping and playing all around us near the Scottish border, we felt thoroughly welcomed by the town and would love to go back again. We even found out it was a favourite destination for L.S.Lowry. We weren't able to take Senna with us on this trip as it would not have been practicable.

In some circumstances it's just too difficult to care for her, as well as assisting Linda.

We wanted to see more of Newcastle but found it difficult to travel around as it's best seen on foot and neither of us can walk very far. We loved it though and I particularly like the fact that a colony of Kittiwakes live under the Tyne Bridge, chattering away to each other, right in the heart of the city.

We couldn't find a suitable place to stay in Newcastle so luckily found the nearby Little Haven hotel at South Shields. I'd never thought that South Shields sounded terribly attractive but that coastline is amazing, and we had a room in which we could watch the ships passing up and down through the mouth of the river Tyne, even while lying in bed - luxury. We slept with the curtains open to see the beautiful sky over the North Sea and the sun coming up, making the ships glow with a variety of beautiful colours and textures. We visited my old friend Viv at Newbiggin, just north of the city, and went south as far as Sunderland and the nearby Angel of the North. We even saw some locations where Vera, the television detective series, is filmed.

Early September brought very sad news, the death of Linda's mum, Olive. She had been very poorly for several years, although not in pain I'm glad to say. Her funeral was at Knebworth on September 5th so we stayed in Welwyn Garden city for a few days before heading home again.

'Olly', as she was known to her dive buddy Sue, was a pioneer of female diving in the UK, at a time when women even had to make their own wetsuits, and was diving long before she and Sue met in the early eighties. They made many trips to the Red

Sea, the Far East, Bali and of course all around the UK. They joined the British Society of Underwater Photographers and went to their monthly meetings in London, and they dived at Swanage, Weymouth and the Farne islands to photograph seals. We have some of her underwater photos on display now.

Later on, we spent a few days in Liverpool in November but yet again found it a bit demanding to get around but had a good time nonetheless, including a night trip on the Mersey Ferry. We had to do both of these particular trips away without Senna, and Danny being at home meant we could leave her in good hands. He went back down south just before Christmas though to be close to his daughter Riley, just in time for Covid to throw a spanner in everyone's works.

Early in 2020 we visited the Idlewild animal sanctuary high up in the hills above Rowen, just south of Conwy. Though Linda found it difficult to move around outside, we stayed and made friends with some of the animals in the office, particularly a pretty little cat called Pippin. Well, Pippin needed a new home and we'd got on so well with him that we agreed to take him on, but almost as soon as we got him home, he started showing his less appealing side and much blood was spilt as he used us for target practice, wow, did he have sharp claws.

We kept him amused as well as we could, even bought him a remote-controlled car for him to chase around, and he wanted for nothing while we just wanted him to stop scratching us to ribbons. Senna was as usual unconcerned about him and vice versa, but we couldn't keep him long term, especially as Linda is on warfarin, and Tanja came to our rescue and found a lovely new home for him with a Rhodesian vet nurse living in Wigan, you don't get many of them to the pound. Caro and Brian have stuck with him and have now moved

Pippin even further away from us
to Scotland.
At last,
we are safe.

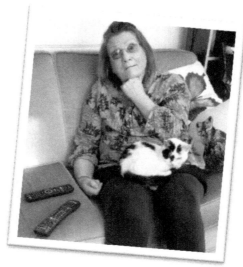

Linda
with
Pippin

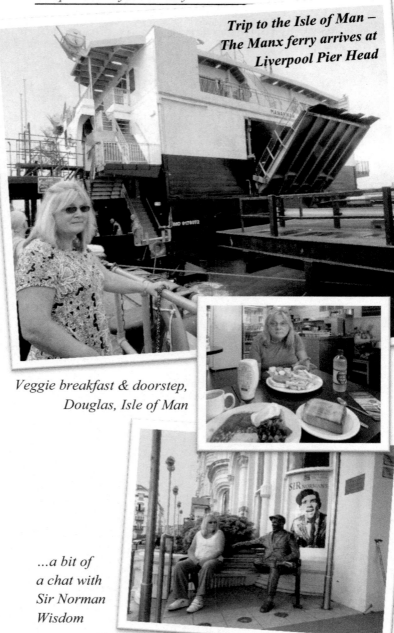

Trip to the Isle of Man – The Manx ferry arrives at Liverpool Pier Head

Veggie breakfast & doorstep, Douglas, Isle of Man

...a bit of a chat with Sir Norman Wisdom

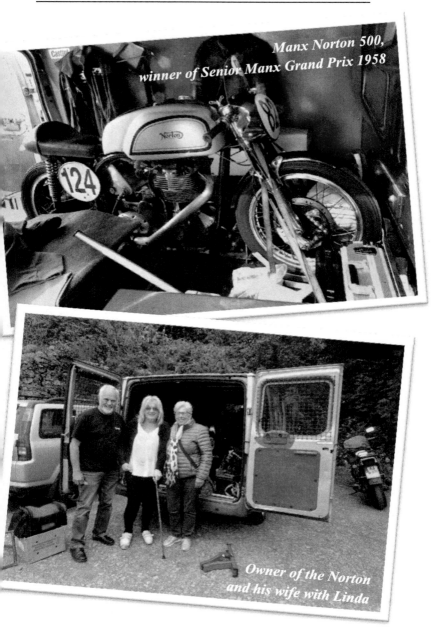

Manx Norton 500, winner of Senior Manx Grand Prix 1958

Owner of the Norton and his wife with Linda

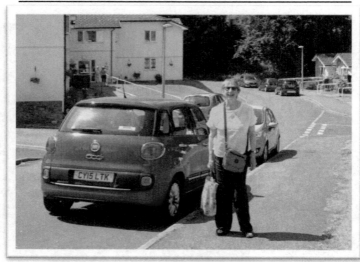

So helpful to Linda, Priscilla
of the Stroke Group

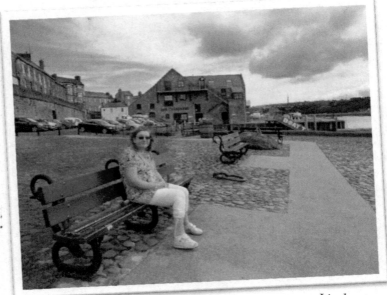

Linda at
beautiful Berwick, Northumberland

CHAPTER 16

DRIVE

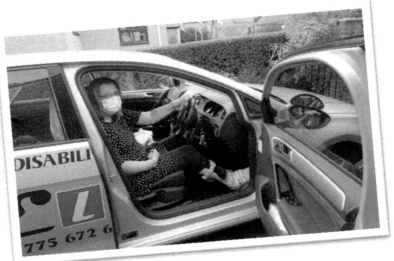

Linda learning to drive again

I don't know when the idea first occurred to us but during the year Linda started taking driving lessons. Oh, she could drive before the stroke, but this would be like starting over. She needed a left foot accelerator, a device on the steering wheel to use left-handed (it's called a lollipop, and has a hub attached with Bluetooth connected buttons to operate lights, indicators, horn, wipers etc.). Of course, it had to be automatic, and we found a wonderful instructor who specialises in teaching disabled people. Elaine was instrumental in getting her ready for her assessment at the Disabled driving centre at Glan Clwyd hospital.

This she passed with flying colours. They were especially impressed that she didn't flap or panic at one point when an incident occurred that many people would have overreacted to. The next step was to obtain her modified licence from the DVLA, who were understandably, due to Covid, operating what I shall politely call a reduced service. What caused even more problems however was the stipulation that the new licence specified a 'modified braking system', even though this meant, according to the driving centre, a modified technique only (i.e. left foot braking).

When we finally decided to get a new car on Motability, my 265 bhp Saab Aero Estate being considered unsuitable for Linda to drive for obvious reasons (also, it only did about 21mpg) we settled on a Toyota Corolla Hatchback hybrid as it was a match for the Saab in terms of performance and it does nearly 50mpg. It's also much nicer to drive than the Saab and very user friendly for Linda.

Motability however chose to interpret 'modified braking system' as something tangible and after a lot of faffing about we had to have a pad fitted to the brake pedal to satisfy the letter of the law.

In the meantime, we were still Saab-ing everywhere, including a trip to Holyhead in

November to see the Sir David Attenborough Polar research ship which was based there undergoing sea trials. We also popped up the road to South Stack but just for the views, the nesting seabirds were long gone by this time.

We weren't sure whether to get one car that we both could drive or a separate car for Linda. The problem with that was that buying a (decent) specific car to suit her, as well as the cost of the necessary adaptations would have probably cost us somewhere between £5,000 and £8,000, and she wouldn't be able to drive a second-hand car to try it out before it was adapted. The pool of cars to choose from in this area is quite small and also, if she was going to drive it on her own, I'd have needed to keep the thirsty Saab going (already fifteen years old and causing problems) or buy a replacement.

We agreed to get one car to share and then wondered whether to buy second hand or go for a Motability car, which meant giving up her relevant share of PIP (Personal Independence Payment) and paying another lump sum up front. Oh, and guess what, not all cars have similar layouts. When looking at used cars, we wondered about a Mercedes A class, but the gear shift is on the right-hand side of the steering column so Linda couldn't reach it. The boot area of the Audi A3 was too small for Senna and the BMW 3 series was too bulky all round.

Also, being a mechanic, you may be surprised to hear that I don't actually like German cars. I think Japanese cars are far superior, and having had two Toyotas in the past (and two Hondas and a Mitsubishi), we looked at the new Corolla Hatchback, a hybrid with a 2-litre petrol engine. It was pretty much perfect for us so we put £3,000 up front and waited until it was ready for collection (it had to be adapted first as well) in July.

It's a lovely car and now that we also have a tracking device, Linda can drive it on her own. In case she hits problems, she only has to press a button to alert me and I can see where she is and go and rescue her, (it even acts as a mobile phone). So far that has not been necessary thank goodness. It's marvellous that she now has a good deal of independence thanks to the car and I have an old Alfa Romeo as a spare in case I need to drive while she's out and about.

With all the limitations that the stroke has imposed on her at last she has some measure of self-determination. It'll never make up for the paralysis and the lack of speech and reading but it has broadened her horizons, especially with lock down behind us. Oh, and it's great to be driven again and see all the things I missed while I had to drive. She's an excellent driver, better than a lot of able-bodied drivers.

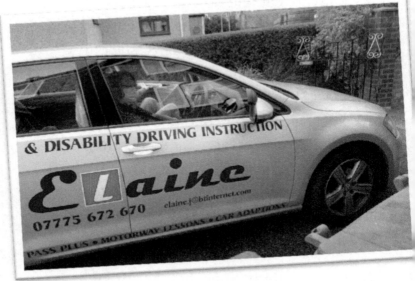

Back on the road!

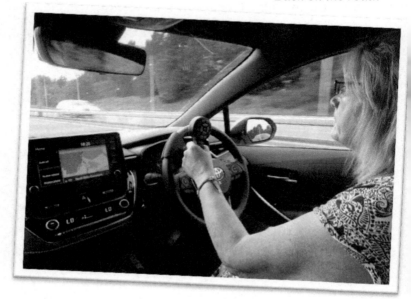

CHAPTER 17

CARRY ON

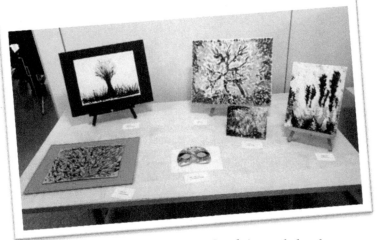

*Linda's work for the
Art Exhibition at Porth Eirias*

Other consequences of the stroke come to mind. One suggestion of an activity for her was photography, but have you ever noticed where the shutter release button is on all cameras? Yup, it's on the right-hand side. Another common problem is trying to get a disabled person through a door in a public building, one that always has a determined door closer attached. Holding the door open with one hand while shepherding your companion through with the other can be surprisingly challenging, especially with a dog in tow as well. A device that would prop the door open for enough time to get through and then switch itself off to allow the door to close would be so useful. I've designed it but getting it made is another matter.

We also like to use sea salt, but in a standard dispenser/grinder one hand needs to hold the container and the other to twist the top, but I found electric salt and pepper grinders that can be held in one hand while a finger presses down a button at the top.

Six batteries and the built-in motor do the rest - marvellous. More jobs for two hands? Zips, fasteners on jewellery, brown paper packages tied up with string... Actually, we did find some bracelets that are tightened with drawstrings, and Linda uses her teeth to pull them tight.

We did go to a knitting class at the 'Lost Sheep Company' shop in Colwyn Bay and Linda tried knitting with one needle, a big fat special one, and when I told the shop owner that Linda only had the use of one hand she said not to worry, she'd get her granddaughter to teach her, a lovely girl of 14 or so, who also has only one hand. I think her disability is due to a birth deformity, but it was a reminder of how our attention can be drawn away from 'normality' and focused on the problems of which we are often unaware that afflict so many people. Volunteering at a spinal injury unit was a sobering experience for me at the age of 40.

Before then I had little idea of the terrible burdens that so many people carry.

Many people rarely come into contact with those who are disabled or seriously ill, and I wonder if society would become kinder and more compassionate if we were all more aware of the suffering of others and were prompted to understand and help those in need. I really think that heightening such awareness should be part of our general education, so often it really is a case of 'there but for the grace of God'.

There are of course many ways that life can become more challenging, such as injury and disease, and many of these arrive out of the blue. A stroke however, specifically damages the brain, from which all movement and expression is controlled, and the effects are usually instant and permanent, a cruel way for the body to turn against itself. Possibly even worse than this though, is when the injury is inflicted deliberately.

Just before Christmas 2021 we stayed at a lovely place called Moggerhanger Park, near Bedford, and one morning there was a craft fair in one of the outbuildings with two sisters in charge of one stall, one of them clearly disabled. It seemed that she had virtually identical disabilities to Linda, but hers were suffered during a domestic assault, and it took years for her to even start to recover from the shock before she could start physical rehabilitation. In the early days of the internet, I used to think that website addresses full of 'slashes' sounded too aggressive and wondered why the word 'stroke', which sounded much gentler, could not be used instead. Sadly, my view of that word has now changed.

Linda used to love researching family history and now has an office in which she can continue her investigations. Clearly, she understands enough of the terms and procedures she needs to and has a laptop to work with. The most impressive recovery she has achieved in the last ten years though must be her ability to drive, it's brought her much needed independence and broadened her horizons so much.

Even this welcome improvement has raised another downside however, as although she goes out on her own, my natural inclination is to ask her about the trip. I might not have been following the route closely and want to ask, and am sure she wants to share with me, where she's gone, what and who she's seen and what she's done. I want to ask if she's seen someone we know, what the traffic was like, if she saw the goats on the Great Orme, or the wild ponies on the Sychnant pass. As with her solo trips to the local, it's pretty much impossible for her to say who was there and what might have happened, it's about as much as we can hope for if she can say how many dogs were in the pub and for me to guess who their owners were.

Being able to speak is the ultimate goal we strive for though, and maybe research is bringing that day nearer. So now we move forward and hope for some improvement in her condition and that all stroke victims can be helped to recover more fully in future.

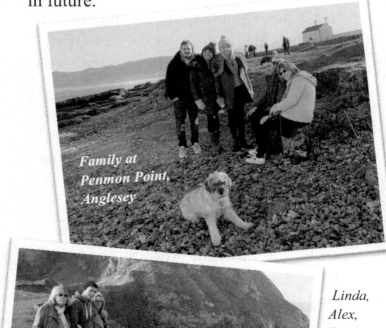

Family at Penmon Point, Anglesey

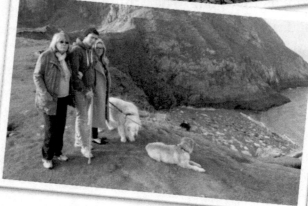

Linda, Alex, Sammy, Billie and Zac – and lots of seals at Angel Bay (Llandudno)

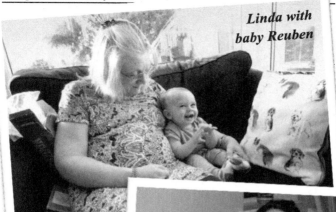

Linda with baby Reuben

Linda with Lois & baby Riley

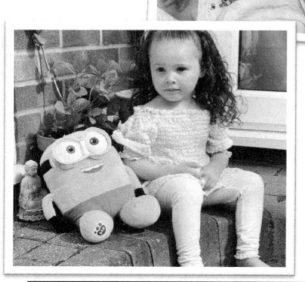

Riley and her little friend

ACKNOWLEDGEMENTS

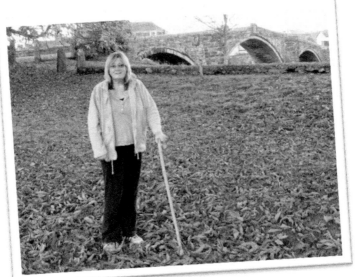

Linda at Llanrwst
(2021)

My grateful thanks go to two special people.

Firstly, to Jamie Robson of Ability.net without whose expert and patient coaching I would have been unable to complete the story successfully, he even compiled the list of contents for me.

Secondly, to Tanja Klein whose graphic design skills were essential in enhancing and positioning the photos and formatting the whole project ready for publication.

Thanks also go to all of those, medical professionals, Stroke group volunteers and friends, who have helped us so much through the last ten years.

In case anyone has not already noticed, all the chapter headings are song titles courtesy of the following musical artistes:

1	*Bohemian like you*	The Dandy Warhols
2	*Let's get together*	Canned Heat
3	*What's going on?*	Marvin Gaye
4	*The shape I'm in*	The Band
5	*Starting over*	John Lennon
6	*Help*	The Beatles
7	*Learning to fly* –	Tom Petty
8	*Get 'em out by Friday*	Genesis
9	*You made me a nervous wreck*	Radio Stars
10	*Ain't no sunshine*	Bill Withers
11	*Let's get married*	The Proclaimers
12	*A design for life*	The Manic Street Preachers
13	*Deeply Dippy*	Right said Fred
14	*I don't wanna talk about it*	Danny Whitten
15	*Synchronicity*	The Police
16	*Drive*	The Cars
17	*Carry on*	Crosby Stills and Nash

Steven Liska

Acknowledgements

Printed in Great Britain
by Amazon